SLOW COOKER CIRRHOSIS DIET COOKBOOK

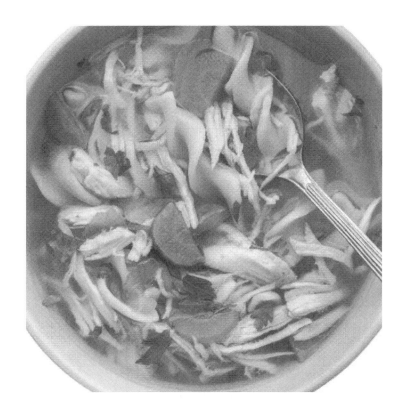

Lysandra Quinn

DISCLAIMER

The content within this book reflects my thoughts, experiences, and beliefs. It is meant for informational and entertainment purposes. While I have taken great care to provide accurate information, I cannot guarantee the absolute correctness or applicability of the content to every individual or situation. Please consult with relevant professionals for advice specific to your needs.

ACKNOWLEDGMENTS

I want to express my deepest gratitude to those who have supported and encouraged me on this creative journey. Your love, patience, and inspiration have been the driving force behind this book. I also thank the talented team of professionals who have contributed their skills to bring this book to life.

TABLE OF CONTENTS

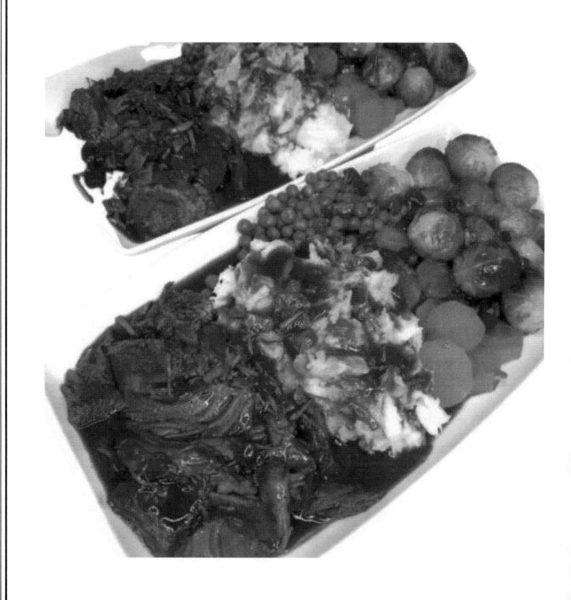

INTRODUCTION

In the quiet, dimly lit room of a hospital, I stood beside my best friend, Emily, who was battling a foe far fiercer than any we had ever encountered. Her eyes, once filled with laughter and vitality, now told a different story. They spoke of pain, exhaustion, and a fear that had taken root deep within her. As a dedicated dietician, I had always believed in the power of food to heal, but never had I witnessed it with such conviction until that fateful day.

Emily had been diagnosed with cirrhosis, a diagnosis that shook our world to its core. Her liver was struggling, and it seemed as though time was slipping through our fingers. The doctors had provided the grim prognosis: a strict diet and a long list of restrictions to manage her condition. And that's when I made a promise to my dearest friend, a promise that would eventually lead to the creation of this cookbook and a journey of healing and hope that I'm excited to share with you.

I vividly remember the moment I told Emily about the slow cooker cirrhosis diet. It was during a gloomy afternoon when the rain was pelting against the windows, mirroring the tears in her eyes. Her once-vibrant spirit seemed to wither with each dietary restriction given by her doctors. It was heart-wrenching to watch her dreams of savouring delicious meals crumble into dust. It was then that I whispered into her ear, "We'll get through this together, and I promise you won't have to give up the joy of eating."

The following weeks were a whirlwind of research, late-night cooking experiments, and unwavering determination. I scoured medical journals and consulted with my colleagues to craft a diet plan that would not only support Emily's liver but also tantalize her taste buds. As a dietician, I knew that flavour and nutrition could coexist, and I was determined to prove it.

One evening, as I was preparing a slow cooker meal for Emily, a transformation began that would forever alter our lives. The aroma of savory herbs and tender cuts of meat wafted through the kitchen, and Emily's eyes widened with curiosity. I ladled a spoonful of the stew into her bowl, and as she took her first bite, something incredible happened. A glimmer of hope sparkled in her eyes, a sparkle I had not seen in a long time. She smiled, and for a moment, the burden of her illness seemed to dissipate.

From that day forward, the slow cooker became our trusted companion in the journey towards Emily's recovery. The gentle, steady cooking process not only preserved the nutritional value of the ingredients but also transformed them into mouthwatering masterpieces that Emily couldn't resist. It was our secret weapon in the fight against cirrhosis, and the effects were nothing short of miraculous.

With each passing week, Emily's strength began to return. She was no longer a frail figure confined to a hospital bed but a determined fighter ready to take on the world. The slow cooker cirrhosis diet was not just about nourishing her body but also feeding her spirit, and it was a testament to the power of the right foods in healing and recovery.

Our journey was marked by ups and downs, but the slow cooker cirrhosis diet became a lifeline for Emily. She thrived on the delicious, liver-friendly meals that I prepared, and her health began to stabilize. We celebrated small victories and milestones that led us to a brighter future. It was in those moments that I knew I had to share our success with others who were facing similar challenges.

This cookbook is the result of our journey—a collection of recipes that saved my best friend's life and transformed our understanding of cirrhosis management. It's a testament to the power of food as medicine, and it's an invitation for you to embark on your own journey of healing and hope. Whether you're a patient, a caregiver, or a concerned friend, this book is a beacon of light in the often-dark world of liver disease.

In the pages that follow, you'll discover a treasure trove of slow cooker recipes specifically designed to support liver health and nourish your body. These recipes are not only delicious but also easy to prepare, making them accessible to anyone, regardless of their culinary expertise. The slow cooker's gentle cooking method ensures that the flavors meld together perfectly, creating meals that will leave your taste buds dancing.

But this cookbook is more than just a collection of recipes; it's a lifeline for those in need, a source of inspiration for those facing adversity, and a symbol of the incredible strength that can be found in the most unexpected places. It's a reminder that we are not alone on this journey and that there is always hope, even in the darkest of times.

So, join us on this journey of healing and hope. Let the recipes in this cookbook become a part of your life, just as they became a part of ours. Together, we can defy the odds and savor the joys of food, even in the face of cirrhosis. Together, we can find strength in each other and in the nourishing power of these slow cooker recipes. Welcome to a new chapter in your life, one filled with delicious meals, renewed hope, and the promise of a healthier tomorrow.

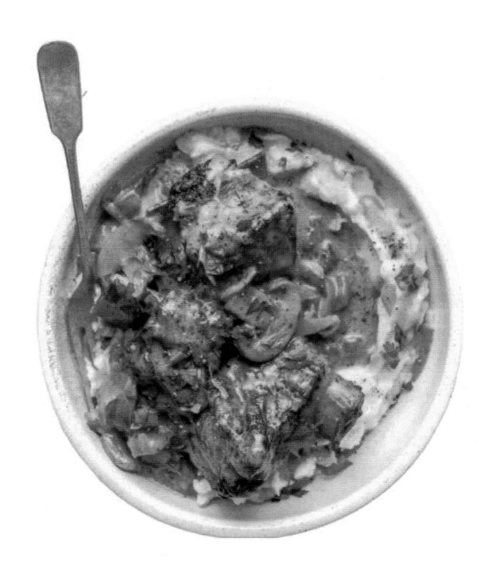

Chapter 1

Welcome to the Slow Cooker Cirrhosis Diet Cookbook

Welcome to the Slow Cooker Cirrhosis Diet Cookbook, a resource designed to help you maintain a healthy and balanced diet while managing cirrhosis. Cirrhosis is a condition that affects the liver, and making the right dietary choices can significantly impact your overall well-being. This cookbook aims to provide you with delicious and nourishing recipes that can be easily prepared in your slow cooker, making meal preparation a breeze.

Understanding Cirrhosis and Diet

Cirrhosis is a condition in which the liver gradually becomes scarred and loses its ability to function properly. It can be caused by various factors, including excessive alcohol consumption, viral infections, or long-term exposure to certain toxins. When dealing with cirrhosis, it is crucial to make dietary choices that support liver health and overall wellness.

A cirrhosis-friendly diet typically includes:

Low Sodium: Cirrhosis can lead to fluid retention, so reducing sodium intake is essential to manage this symptom.

Adequate Protein: While your liver may have trouble processing proteins, it's important to maintain a healthy protein intake to support muscle strength and overall health.

Healthy Fats: Choosing good fats, such as those found in avocados, nuts, and olive oil, can help protect your liver.

Small, Frequent Meals: Eating smaller meals throughout the day can help your liver process nutrients more effectively.

Vitamins and Minerals: Ensure you get enough vitamins and minerals, especially vitamin D, vitamin K, and calcium, which can be affected by cirrhosis.

Using Your Slow Cooker for Healthy Cooking

A slow cooker is a fantastic tool for preparing nutritious meals that align with a cirrhosis-friendly diet. Here are some reasons why using a slow cooker can benefit you:

Convenience: Slow cookers are incredibly easy to use. You can prepare your ingredients in the morning, set the cooker, and come home to a delicious, ready-to-eat meal.

Flavor: Slow cooking allows flavors to meld and intensify, resulting in savory and mouthwatering dishes.

Nutrient Retention: Slow cooking at lower temperatures helps preserve the nutritional value of your ingredients.

Tenderization: Tough cuts of meat can become tender and flavorful when cooked slowly in a crockpot.

In this cookbook, you'll find a variety of cirrhosis-friendly recipes that are specifically tailored for your slow cooker. These recipes focus on using ingredients that support liver health and offer you a delightful culinary experience. Whether you're in the early stages of cirrhosis or further along in your journey, this cookbook is designed to help you make the most of your meals while promoting your overall well-being.

We hope you find the Slow Cooker Cirrhosis Diet Cookbook a valuable resource on your path to better health. Enjoy the culinary journey and remember that making mindful food choices can have a positive impact on your liver health.

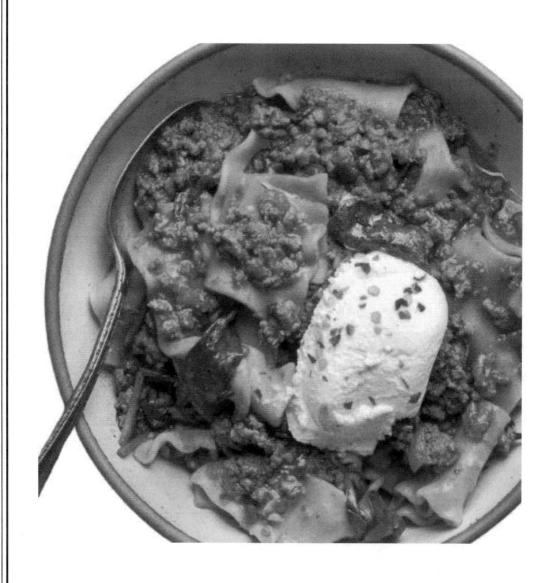

Chapter 2

Breakfasts and Brunches

Slow Cooker Oatmeal

Cooking Time: 4 hours

Serving: 4

Ingredients:

- ✓ 1 cup steel-cut oats
- ✓ 4 cups low-fat milk
- ✓ 1/4 cup honey
- ✓ 1/4 teaspoon salt
- ✓ 1/2 cup chopped fresh fruit (e.g., apples or berries)

Instructions:

1. Combine oats, milk, honey, and salt in the slow cooker.
2. Cook on low for 4 hours.
3. Serve topped with fresh fruit.

Nutritional Information (per serving):

Calories: 250, Protein: 9g, Carbs: 45g, Fat: 4g, Fiber: 5g.

Veggie Frittata

Cooking Time: 3 hours

Serving: 6

Ingredients:

- ✓ 8 large eggs
- ✓ 1/2 cup skim milk
- ✓ 1 cup diced bell peppers, onions, and spinach,
- ✓ 1/2 cup low-fat cheese
- ✓ Salt and pepper to taste

Instructions:

1. Whisk eggs and milk in a bowl.
2. Grease the slow cooker and add veggies.
3. Pour egg mixture over veggies and sprinkle with cheese.
4. Cook on low for 3 hours.

Nutritional Information (per serving):

Calories: 160, Protein: 13g, Carbs: 4g, Fat: 10g.

Slow Cooker Quinoa Porridge

Cooking Time: 2 hours

Serving: 4

Ingredients:

- ✓ 1 cup quinoa, rinsed.
- ✓ 2 cups low-fat coconut milk
- ✓ 1/4 cup raisins
- ✓ 1/4 teaspoon cinnamon
- ✓ 1 tablespoon honey

Instructions:

1. Combine quinoa, coconut milk, raisins, and cinnamon in the slow cooker.
2. Cook on low for 2 hours.
3. Drizzle with honey before serving.

Nutritional Information (per serving):

Calories: 250, Protein: 6g, Carbs: 44g, Fat: 6g, Fiber: 3g.

Crock-Pot Apple Cinnamon Oatmeal

Cooking Time: 6 hours

Serving: 6

Ingredients:

- ✓ 2 cups steel-cut oats
- ✓ 8 cups low-fat milk
- ✓ 2 apples peeled and chopped.
- ✓ 2 teaspoons cinnamon
- ✓ 1/4 cup maple syrup

Instructions:

1. Combine oats, milk, apples, cinnamon, and maple syrup in the slow cooker.
2. Cook on low for 6 hours.

Nutritional Information (per serving):

Calories: 300, Protein: 12g, Carbs: 50g, Fat: 6g, Fiber: 7g.

Slow Cooker Breakfast Burritos

Cooking Time: 4 hours

Serving: 4

Ingredients:

- ✓ 8 eggs
- ✓ 1/2 cup diced tomatoes and bell peppers.
- ✓ 1/2 cup cooked turkey sausage
- ✓ 1/4 cup low-fat cheese
- ✓ Whole-wheat tortillas

Instructions:

1. Whisk eggs and pour them into the greased slow cooker.
2. Add tomatoes, bell peppers, sausage, and cheese.
3. Cook on low for 4 hours.
4. Serve in whole-wheat tortillas.

Nutritional Information (per serving):

Calories: 300, Protein: 20g, Carbs: 20g, Fat: 15g.

Slow Cooker Egg and Vegetable Casserole

Cooking Time: 3 hours

Serving: 6

Ingredients:

- ✓ 8 eggs
- ✓ 1 cup diced zucchini, mushrooms, and spinach.
- ✓ 1/2 cup low-fat cheese
- ✓ Salt and pepper to taste

Instructions:

1. Whisk eggs and pour them into the greased slow cooker.
2. Add veggies and cheese.
3. Cook on low for 3 hours.

Nutritional Information (per serving):

Calories: 150, Protein: 14g, Carbs: 5g, Fat: 8g.

Slow Cooker Breakfast Quiche

Cooking Time: 4 hours

Serving: 6

Ingredients:

- ✓ 6 large eggs
- ✓ 1/2 cup low-fat milk
- ✓ 1 cup diced ham.
- ✓ 1/2 cup diced bell peppers and onions.
- ✓ 1/2 cup low-fat cheese
- ✓ Salt and pepper to taste

Instructions:

1. Whisk eggs and milk in a bowl.
2. Grease the slow cooker and add ham, peppers, onions, and cheese.
3. Pour egg mixture over ingredients.
4. Cook on low for 4 hours.

Nutritional Information (per serving):

Calories: 220, Protein: 18g, Carbs: 5g, Fat: 13g.

Crock-Pot Banana Nut Bread Oatmeal

Cooking Time: 4 hours

Serving: 4

Ingredients:

- ✓ 1 cup steel-cut oats
- ✓ 4 cups low-fat milk
- ✓ 2 ripe bananas, mashed.
- ✓ 1/4 cup chopped nuts.
- ✓ 1/4 cup honey

Instructions:

1. Combine oats, milk, mashed bananas, nuts, and honey in the slow cooker.
2. Cook on low for 4 hours.

Nutritional Information (per serving):

Calories: 280, Protein: 9g, Carbs: 46g, Fat: 8g, Fiber: 6g.

Slow Cooker Greek Yogurt Parfait

Cooking Time: 2 hours

Serving: 4

Ingredients:

- ✓ 2 cups low-fat Greek yogurt
- ✓ 1/4 cup honey
- ✓ 1 cup mixed berries
- ✓ 1/4 cup granola

Instructions:

1. Mix Greek yogurt and honey in the slow cooker.
2. Cook on low for 2 hours.
3. Serve topped with mixed berries and granola.

Nutritional Information (per serving):

Calories: 220, Protein: 16g, Carbs: 35g, Fat: 2g.

Slow Cooker Chia Seed Pudding

Cooking Time: 2 hours

Serving: 4

Ingredients:

- ✓ 1/2 cup chia seeds
- ✓ 2 cups low-fat almond milk
- ✓ 1/4 cup maple syrup
- ✓ 1/2 teaspoon vanilla extract
- ✓ Sliced fruit for topping

Instructions:

1. Combine chia seeds, almond milk, maple syrup, and vanilla extract in the slow cooker.
2. Cook on low for 2 hours, stirring occasionally.
3. Chill in the refrigerator for a few hours or overnight.
4. Serve with sliced fruit on top.

Nutritional Information (per serving):

Calories: 180, Protein: 4g, Carbs: 25g, Fat: 7g, Fiber: 10g.

Chapter 3

Hearty Soups and Stews

Slow Cooker Chicken and Rice Soup

Cooking Time: 4 hours

Serving: 6

Ingredients:

- ✓ 1-pound boneless, skinless chicken breasts
- ✓ 1 cup white rice
- ✓ 4 cups low-sodium chicken broth
- ✓ 2 carrots, chopped.
- ✓ 2 celery stalks, chopped.
- ✓ 1 onion, diced.
- ✓ 2 cloves garlic, minced.
- ✓ Salt and pepper to taste

Instructions:

1. Place chicken, rice, vegetables, and broth in the slow cooker.
2. Cook on low for 4 hours.
3. Shred the chicken, season with salt and pepper, and serve.

Nutritional Information (per serving):

Calories: 250, Protein: 20g, Carbs: 30g, Fat: 4g, Fiber: 2g.

Slow Cooker Lentil Stew

Cooking Time: 6 hours

Serving: 6

Ingredients:

- ✓ 1 cup dried green or brown lentils, rinsed.
- ✓ 4 cups low-sodium vegetable broth
- ✓ 2 carrots, chopped.
- ✓ 2 celery stalks, chopped.
- ✓ 1 onion, diced.
- ✓ 2 cloves garlic, minced.
- ✓ 1 teaspoon cumin
- ✓ 1/2 teaspoon paprika
- ✓ Salt and pepper to taste

Instructions:

1. Combine all ingredients in the slow cooker.
2. Cook on low for 6 hours.
3. Season with salt and pepper before serving.

Nutritional Information (per serving):

Calories: 220, Protein: 12g, Carbs: 35g, Fat: 2g, Fiber: 11g.

Slow Cooker Vegetable Barley Soup

Cooking Time: 4 hours

Serving: 6

Ingredients:

- ✓ 1 cup pearl barley
- ✓ 4 cups low-sodium vegetable broth
- ✓ 2 carrots, chopped.
- ✓ 2 celery stalks, chopped.
- ✓ 1 onion, diced.
- ✓ 2 cloves garlic, minced.
- ✓ 1 cup mixed vegetables (corn, peas, green beans)
- ✓ Salt and pepper to taste

Instructions:

1. Combine barley, vegetables, and broth in the slow cooker.
2. Cook on low for 4 hours.
3. Season with salt and pepper before serving.

Nutritional Information (per serving):

Calories: 220, Protein: 6g, Carbs: 45g, Fat: 1g, Fiber: 10g.

Slow Cooker Beef and Vegetable Stew

Cooking Time: 6 hours

Serving: 6

Ingredients:

- ✓ 1-pound lean beef stew meat
- ✓ 4 cups low-sodium beef broth
- ✓ 2 potatoes, chopped.
- ✓ 2 carrots, chopped.
- ✓ 1 onion, diced.
- ✓ 2 cloves garlic, minced.
- ✓ 1 teaspoon thyme
- ✓ Salt and pepper to taste

Instructions:

1. Combine beef, vegetables, broth, and spices in the slow cooker.
2. Cook on low for 6 hours.
3. Season with salt and pepper before serving.

Nutritional Information (per serving):

Calories: 250, Protein: 20g, Carbs: 20g, Fat: 8g, Fiber: 4g.

Slow Cooker Split Pea Soup

Cooking Time: 8 hours

Serving: 6

Ingredients:

- ✓ 1 cup dried split peas, rinsed.
- ✓ 4 cups low-sodium vegetable broth
- ✓ 2 carrots, chopped.
- ✓ 2 celery stalks, chopped.
- ✓ 1 onion, diced.
- ✓ 2 cloves garlic, minced.
- ✓ 1 bay leaf
- ✓ Salt and pepper to taste

Instructions:

1. Combine split peas, vegetables, broth, and bay leaf in the slow cooker.
2. Cook on low for 8 hours.
3. Remove the bay leaf, season with salt and pepper, and serve.

Nutritional Information (per serving):

Calories: 180, Protein: 10g, Carbs: 30g, Fat: 1g, Fiber: 10g.

Slow Cooker Minestrone Soup

Cooking Time: 4 hours

Serving: 6

Ingredients:

- ✓ 1 cup small pasta (e.g., ditalini)
- ✓ 4 cups low-sodium vegetable broth
- ✓ 2 carrots, chopped.
- ✓ 2 celery stalks, chopped.
- ✓ 1 onion, diced.
- ✓ 2 cloves garlic, minced.
- ✓ 1 can (15 oz) diced tomatoes.
- ✓ 1 can (15 oz) kidney beans, drained
- ✓ 1 teaspoon Italian seasoning
- ✓ Salt and pepper to taste

Instructions:

1. Combine pasta, vegetables, broth, tomatoes, beans, and spices in the slow cooker.
2. Cook on low for 4 hours.
3. Season with salt and pepper before serving.

Nutritional Information (per serving):

Calories: 250, Protein: 9g, Carbs: 50g, Fat: 2g, Fiber: 8g.

Slow Cooker Turkey and Vegetable Chili

Cooking Time: 6 hours

Serving: 6

Ingredients:

- ✓ 1 pound ground turkey
- ✓ 2 cans (15 oz each) low-sodium kidney beans, drained
- ✓ 1 can (15 oz) diced tomatoes.
- ✓ 2 bell peppers, diced.
- ✓ 1 onion, diced.
- ✓ 2 cloves garlic, minced.
- ✓ 2 tablespoons chili powder
- ✓ Salt and pepper to taste

Instructions:

1. Brown the ground turkey in a pan and drain excess fat.
2. Add turkey, vegetables, beans, tomatoes, and spices to the slow cooker.
3. Cook on low for 6 hours.
4. Season with salt and pepper before serving.

Nutritional Information (per serving):

Calories: 290, Protein: 20g, Carbs: 40g, Fat: 6g, Fiber: 10g.

Slow Cooker Mushroom and Barley Stew

Cooking Time: 5 hours

Serving: 6

Ingredients:

- ✓ 1 cup pearl barley
- ✓ 4 cups low-sodium vegetable broth
- ✓ 1-pound mushrooms, sliced
- ✓ 2 carrots, chopped.
- ✓ 2 celery stalks, chopped.
- ✓ 1 onion, diced.
- ✓ 2 cloves garlic, minced.
- ✓ 1 teaspoon thyme
- ✓ Salt and pepper to taste

Instructions:

1. Combine barley, mushrooms, vegetables, broth, and spices in the slow cooker.
2. Cook on low for 5 hours.
3. Season with salt and pepper before serving.

Nutritional Information (per serving):

Calories: 240, Protein: 7g, Carbs: 50g, Fat: 1g, Fiber: 9g.

Slow Cooker Potato Leek Soup

Cooking Time: 4 hours

Serving: 6

Ingredients:

- ✓ 4 large potatoes peeled and chopped.
- ✓ 3 leeks, chopped (white and light green parts)
- ✓ 4 cups low-sodium vegetable broth
- ✓ 2 cloves garlic, minced.
- ✓ 1/2 cup low-fat Greek yogurt
- ✓ Salt and pepper to taste

Instructions:

1. Combine potatoes, leeks, broth, and garlic in the slow cooker.
2. Cook on low for 4 hours.
3. Use an immersion blender to blend until smooth, then stir in Greek yogurt.
4. Season with salt and pepper before serving.

Nutritional Information (per serving):

Calories: 180, Protein: 4g, Carbs: 40g, Fat: 1g, Fiber: 5g.

Slow Cooker Black Bean and Sweet Potato Stew

Cooking Time: 5 hours

Serving: 6

Ingredients:

- ✓ 2 sweet potatoes peeled and chopped.
- ✓ 2 cans (15 oz each) black beans, drained and rinsed.
- ✓ 2 bell peppers, diced.
- ✓ 1 onion, diced.
- ✓ 2 cloves garlic, minced.
- ✓ 1 teaspoon cumin
- ✓ 1/2 teaspoon chili powder
- ✓ Salt and pepper to taste

Instructions:

1. Combine sweet potatoes, beans, vegetables, and spices in the slow cooker.
2. Cook on low for 5 hours.
3. Season with salt and pepper before serving.

Nutritional Information (per serving):

Calories: 220, Protein: 8g, Carbs: 45g, Fat: 1g, Fiber: 10g.

Chapter 4

Nutrient-Rich Entrees

Slow Cooker Lemon Herb Chicken

Cooking Time: 4 hours

Serving: 4

Ingredients:

- ✓ 4 boneless, skinless chicken breasts
- ✓ 1 lemon juiced and zested.
- ✓ 1/4 cup low-sodium chicken broth
- ✓ 2 cloves garlic, minced.
- ✓ 1 teaspoon dried thyme
- ✓ Salt and pepper to taste

Instructions:

1. Place chicken in the slow cooker.
2. In a bowl, mix lemon juice, zest, chicken broth, garlic, thyme, salt, and pepper.
3. Pour the mixture over the chicken.
4. Cook on low for 4 hours.

Nutritional Information (per serving):

Calories: 190, Protein: 30g, Carbs: 2g, Fat: 7g, Fiber: 1g.

Slow Cooker Turkey and Vegetable Curry

Cooking Time: 6 hours

Serving: 6

Ingredients:

- ✓ 1-pound lean ground turkey
- ✓ 2 cups diced sweet potatoes.
- ✓ 2 cups cauliflower florets
- ✓ 1 can (15 oz) chickpeas, drained
- ✓ 1 onion, diced.
- ✓ 2 cloves garlic, minced.
- ✓ 1 can (15 oz) low-sodium tomato sauce
- ✓ 2 tablespoons curry powder
- ✓ Salt and pepper to taste

Instructions:

1. Brown turkey in a pan and drain excess fat.
2. Add turkey, vegetables, chickpeas, tomato sauce, curry powder, salt, and pepper to the slow cooker.
3. Cook on low for 6 hours.

Nutritional Information (per serving):

Calories: 280, Protein: 18g, Carbs: 38g, Fat: 6g, Fiber: 10g.

Slow Cooker Salmon with Dill Sauce

Cooking Time: 3 hours

Serving: 4

Ingredients:

- ✓ 4 salmon fillets
- ✓ 1/4 cup low-fat Greek yogurt
- ✓ 1/4 cup fresh dill, chopped.
- ✓ 1 lemon juiced and zested.
- ✓ 2 cloves garlic, minced.
- ✓ Salt and pepper to taste

Instructions:

1. Place salmon in the slow cooker.
2. In a bowl, mix yogurt, dill, lemon juice, zest, garlic, salt, and pepper.
3. Spread the mixture over the salmon.
4. Cook on low for 3 hours.

Nutritional Information (per serving):

Calories: 280, Protein: 30g, Carbs: 4g, Fat: 15g, Fiber: 1g.

Slow Cooker Lentil and Spinach Stew

Cooking Time: 5 hours

Serving: 6

Ingredients:

- ✓ 1 cup brown or green lentils, rinsed.
- ✓ 4 cups low-sodium vegetable broth
- ✓ 2 carrots, chopped.
- ✓ 2 celery stalks, chopped.
- ✓ 1 onion, diced.
- ✓ 2 cloves garlic, minced.
- ✓ 4 cups fresh spinach
- ✓ 1 teaspoon cumin
- ✓ Salt and pepper to taste

Instructions:

1. Combine lentils, vegetables, broth, cumin, salt, and pepper in the slow cooker.
2. Cook on low for 5 hours.
3. Stir in fresh spinach just before serving.

Nutritional Information (per serving):

Calories: 220, Protein: 12g, Carbs: 40g, Fat: 1g, Fiber: 10g.

Slow Cooker Quinoa and Black Bean Casserole

Cooking Time: 4 hours

Serving: 6

Ingredients:

- ✓ 1 cup quinoa, rinsed.
- ✓ 2 cans (15 oz each) low-sodium black beans, drained
- ✓ 1 can (15 oz) diced tomatoes.
- ✓ 1 bell pepper, diced.
- ✓ 1 onion, diced.
- ✓ 2 cloves garlic, minced.
- ✓ 1 teaspoon chili powder
- ✓ Salt and pepper to taste

Instructions:

1. Combine quinoa, beans, vegetables, tomatoes, chili powder, salt, and pepper in the slow cooker.
2. Cook on low for 4 hours.

Nutritional Information (per serving):

Calories: 250, Protein: 12g, Carbs: 45g, Fat: 2g, Fiber: 10g.

Slow Cooker Beef and Vegetable Stir-Fry

Cooking Time: 5 hours

Serving: 6

Ingredients:

- ✓ 1-pound lean beef stew meat
- ✓ 2 cups broccoli florets
- ✓ 2 cups snap peas
- ✓ 1 red bell pepper, sliced.
- ✓ 1 onion, sliced.
- ✓ 1/4 cup low-sodium soy sauce
- ✓ 2 cloves garlic, minced.
- ✓ 1 teaspoon ginger, minced.
- ✓ 1 tablespoon honey
- ✓ Salt and pepper to taste

Instructions:

1. Place beef, vegetables, soy sauce, garlic, ginger, honey, salt, and pepper in the slow cooker.
2. Cook on low for 5 hours.

Nutritional Information (per serving):

Calories: 280, Protein: 25g, Carbs: 20g, Fat: 10g, Fiber: 6g.

Slow Cooker Tofu and Vegetable Curry

Cooking Time: 4 hours

Serving: 4

Ingredients:

- ✓ 1 block (14 oz) extra-firm tofu, cubed.
- ✓ 2 cups broccoli florets
- ✓ 1 cup sliced carrots.
- ✓ 1 can (15 oz) chickpeas, drained
- ✓ 1 onion, diced.
- ✓ 2 cloves garlic, minced.
- ✓ 1 can (15 oz) low-sodium tomato sauce
- ✓ 2 tablespoons curry powder
- ✓ Salt and pepper to taste

Instructions:

1. Combine tofu, vegetables, chickpeas, tomato sauce, curry powder, salt, and pepper in the slow cooker.
2. Cook on low for 4 hours.

Nutritional Information (per serving):

Calories: 250, Protein: 18g, Carbs: 30g, Fat: 10g, Fiber: 9g.

Slow Cooker Vegetable and Quinoa Stuffed Peppers

Cooking Time: 4 hours

Serving: 4

Ingredients:

- ✓ 4 bell peppers, tops removed, and seeds removed.
- ✓ 1 cup quinoa, rinsed.
- ✓ 2 cups low-sodium vegetable broth
- ✓ 1 can (15 oz) black beans, drained
- ✓ 1 cup corn kernels
- ✓ 1 onion, diced.
- ✓ 2 cloves garlic, minced.
- ✓ 1 teaspoon chili powder
- ✓ Salt and pepper to taste

Instructions:

1. Place the hollowed peppers in the slow cooker.
2. In a bowl, mix quinoa, broth, beans, corn, onion, garlic, chili powder, salt, and pepper.
3. Fill peppers with the quinoa mixture.
4. Cook on low for 4 hours.

Nutritional Information (per serving):

Calories: 350, Protein: 14g, Carbs: 70g, Fat: 3g, Fiber: 10g.

Slow Cooker Teriyaki Chicken and Vegetables

Cooking Time: 4 hours

Serving: 4

Ingredients:

- ✓ 4 boneless, skinless chicken breasts
- ✓ 2 cups broccoli florets
- ✓ 1 red bell pepper, sliced.
- ✓ 1 yellow bell pepper, sliced.
- ✓ 1/2 cup low-sodium teriyaki sauce
- ✓ 2 cloves garlic, minced.
- ✓ Salt and pepper to taste

Instructions:

1. Place chicken, vegetables, teriyaki sauce, garlic, salt, and pepper in the slow cooker.
2. Cook on low for 4 hours.

Nutritional Information (per serving):

Calories: 270, Protein: 30g, Carbs: 20g, Fat: 6g, Fiber: 4g.

Slow Cooker Sweet Potato and Black Bean Chili

Cooking Time: 6 hours

Serving: 6

Ingredients:

- ✓ 2 sweet potatoes peeled and chopped.
- ✓ 2 cans (15 oz each) black beans, drained
- ✓ 1 can (15 oz) diced tomatoes.
- ✓ 1 onion, diced.
- ✓ 2 cloves garlic, minced.
- ✓ 2 teaspoons chili powder
- ✓ 1/2 teaspoon cumin
- ✓ Salt and pepper to taste

Instructions:

1. Combine sweet potatoes, beans, tomatoes, onion, garlic, chili powder, cumin, salt, and pepper in the slow cooker.
2. Cook on low for 6 hours.

Nutritional Information (per serving):

Calories: 250, Protein: 10g, Carbs: 50g, Fat: 1g, Fiber: 12g.

Chapter 5

Side Dishes and Vegetables

Slow Cooker Mashed Potatoes

Cooking Time: 4 hours

Serving: 6

Ingredients:

- ✓ 6 large potatoes peeled and cubed.
- ✓ 2 cloves garlic, minced.
- ✓ 1/2 cup low-fat milk
- ✓ 2 tablespoons low-fat butter or margarine
- ✓ Salt and pepper to taste

Instructions:

1. Place potatoes and garlic in the slow cooker.
2. Cook on low for 4 hours.
3. Mash the potatoes, add milk, butter, salt, and pepper.

Nutritional Information (per serving):

Calories: 180, Protein: 4g, Carbs: 35g, Fat: 2g, Fiber: 3g.

Slow Cooker Lemon Garlic Asparagus

Cooking Time: 2 hours

Serving: 4

Ingredients:

- ✓ 1 bunch asparagus, trimmed.
- ✓ 2 cloves garlic, minced.
- ✓ 1 lemon zested and juiced.
- ✓ 2 tablespoons olive oil
- ✓ Salt and pepper to taste

Instructions:

1. Place asparagus in the slow cooker.
2. In a bowl, mix garlic, lemon juice, lemon zest, olive oil, salt, and pepper.
3. Pour the mixture over the asparagus.
4. Cook on low for 2 hours.

Nutritional Information (per serving):

Calories: 60, Protein: 2g, Carbs: 4g, Fat: 5g, Fiber: 2g.

Slow Cooker Brown Sugar Glazed Carrots

Cooking Time: 3 hours

Serving: 4

Ingredients:

- ✓ 1 pound baby carrots
- ✓ 1/4 cup brown sugar
- ✓ 2 tablespoons low-fat butter or margarine
- ✓ 1/2 teaspoon ground cinnamon
- ✓ Salt to taste

Instructions:

1. Place carrots in the slow cooker.
2. In a bowl, mix brown sugar, butter, cinnamon, and salt.
3. Pour the mixture over the carrots.
4. Cook on low for 3 hours.

Nutritional Information (per serving):

Calories: 120, Protein: 1g, Carbs: 24g, Fat: 3g, Fiber: 3g.

Slow Cooker Quinoa Pilaf with Vegetables

Cooking Time: 2 hours

Serving: 6

Ingredients:

- ✓ 1 cup quinoa, rinsed.
- ✓ 2 cups low-sodium vegetable broth
- ✓ 1 cup mixed vegetables (peas, carrots, corn)
- ✓ 1 onion, diced.
- ✓ 2 cloves garlic, minced.
- ✓ 1/4 cup chopped fresh parsley.
- ✓ Salt and pepper to taste

Instructions:

1. Place quinoa, vegetables, broth, onion, garlic, parsley, salt, and pepper in the slow cooker.
2. Cook on low for 2 hours.

Nutritional Information (per serving):

Calories: 150, Protein: 5g, Carbs: 30g, Fat: 1g, Fiber: 4g.

Slow Cooker Cinnamon Apples

Cooking Time: 2 hours

Serving: 4

Ingredients:

- ✓ 4 apples cored and sliced.
- ✓ 1/4 cup brown sugar
- ✓ 1 teaspoon ground cinnamon
- ✓ 1/4 cup low-fat butter or margarine
- ✓ Instructions:
- ✓ Place apples in the slow cooker.
- ✓ In a bowl, mix brown sugar, cinnamon, and butter.
- ✓ Pour the mixture over the apples.
- ✓ Cook on low for 2 hours.

Nutritional Information (per serving):

Calories: 140, Protein: 1g, Carbs: 30g, Fat: 2g, Fiber: 4g.

Slow Cooker Roasted Garlic Mushrooms

Cooking Time: 3 hours

Serving: 4

Ingredients:

- ✓ 1-pound mushrooms, cleaned and halved
- ✓ 4 cloves garlic, minced.
- ✓ 2 tablespoons olive oil
- ✓ 1/4 cup fresh parsley, chopped.
- ✓ Salt and pepper to taste

Instructions:

1. Place mushrooms in the slow cooker.
2. In a bowl, mix garlic, olive oil, parsley, salt, and pepper.
3. Pour the mixture over the mushrooms.
4. Cook on low for 3 hours.

Nutritional Information (per serving):

Calories: 90, Protein: 3g, Carbs: 6g, Fat: 6g, Fiber: 2g.

Slow Cooker Garlic Herb Potatoes

Cooking Time: 3 hours

Serving: 4

Ingredients:

- ✓ 1 pound baby potatoes, halved.
- ✓ 4 cloves garlic, minced.
- ✓ 2 tablespoons olive oil
- ✓ 1 teaspoon dried rosemary
- ✓ 1 teaspoon dried thyme
- ✓ Salt and pepper to taste

Instructions:

1. Place potatoes in the slow cooker.
2. In a bowl, mix garlic, olive oil, rosemary, thyme, salt, and pepper.
3. Pour the mixture over the potatoes.
4. Cook on low for 3 hours.

Nutritional Information (per serving):

Calories: 150, Protein: 2g, Carbs: 20g, Fat: 7g, Fiber: 2g.

Slow Cooker Maple Glazed Butternut Squash

Cooking Time: 4 hours

Serving: 6

Ingredients:

- ✓ 1 butternut squash peeled and cubed.
- ✓ 1/4 cup pure maple syrup
- ✓ 2 tablespoons low-fat butter or margarine
- ✓ 1/2 teaspoon ground cinnamon
- ✓ Salt and pepper to taste

Instructions:

1. Place butternut squash in the slow cooker.
2. In a bowl, mix maple syrup, butter, cinnamon, salt, and pepper.
3. Pour the mixture over the squash.
4. Cook on low for 4 hours.

Nutritional Information (per serving):

Calories: 150, Protein: 2g, Carbs: 35g, Fat: 2g, Fiber: 4g.

Slow Cooker Balsamic Glazed Brussels Sprouts

Cooking Time: 3 hours

Serving: 4

Ingredients:

- ✓ 1 pound Brussels sprouts trimmed and halved.
- ✓ 2 tablespoons balsamic vinegar
- ✓ 2 tablespoons olive oil
- ✓ 2 cloves garlic, minced.
- ✓ Salt and pepper to taste

Instructions:

1. Place Brussels sprouts in the slow cooker.
2. In a bowl, mix balsamic vinegar, olive oil, garlic, salt, and pepper.
3. Pour the mixture over the Brussels sprouts.
4. Cook on low for 3 hours.

Nutritional Information (per serving):

Calories: 90, Protein: 3g, Carbs: 10g, Fat: 5g, Fiber: 4g.

Slow Cooker Wild Rice and Mushroom Pilaf

Cooking Time: 4 hours

Serving: 6

Ingredients:

- ✓ 1 cup wild rice
- ✓ 4 cups low-sodium vegetable broth
- ✓ 1-pound mushrooms, sliced
- ✓ 1 onion, diced.
- ✓ 2 cloves garlic, minced.
- ✓ 1/4 cup fresh parsley, chopped.
- ✓ Salt and pepper to taste

Instructions:

1. Place wild rice, broth, mushrooms, onion, garlic, parsley, salt, and pepper in the slow cooker.
2. Cook on low for 4 hours.

Nutritional Information (per serving):

Calories: 180, Protein: 6g, Carbs: 30g, Fat: 4g, Fiber: 4g.

Chapter 6

Snacks and Appetizers

Slow Cooker Spinach and Artichoke Dip

Cooking Time: 2 hours

Serving: 8

Ingredients:

- ✓ 1 cup frozen spinach thawed and drained.
- ✓ 1 can (14 oz) artichoke hearts, drained and chopped.
- ✓ 1 cup low-fat Greek yogurt
- ✓ 1 cup light cream cheese
- ✓ 1/2 cup grated Parmesan cheese
- ✓ 1/2 cup low-fat mozzarella cheese
- ✓ 2 cloves garlic, minced.
- ✓ Salt and pepper to taste

Instructions:

1. Combine all ingredients in the slow cooker.
2. Cook on low for 2 hours, stirring occasionally.

Nutritional Information (per serving):

Calories: 180, Protein: 10g, Carbs: 6g, Fat: 14g, Fiber: 2g.

Slow Cooker Salsa Verde Chicken Wings

Cooking Time: 3 hours

Serving: 6

Ingredients:

- ✓ 2 pounds chicken wings
- ✓ 1 cup salsa Verde
- ✓ 2 cloves garlic, minced.
- ✓ 1 teaspoon cumin
- ✓ Salt and pepper to taste

Instructions:

1. Place chicken wings in the slow cooker.
2. In a bowl, mix salsa Verde, garlic, cumin, salt, and pepper.
3. Pour the mixture over the chicken wings.
4. Cook on low for 3 hours.

Nutritional Information (per serving):

Calories: 220, Protein: 20g, Carbs: 4g, Fat: 14g, Fiber: 1g.

Slow Cooker Roasted Red Pepper Hummus

Cooking Time: 2 hours

Serving: 8

Ingredients:

- ✓ 1 can (15 oz) chickpeas, drained
- ✓ 1/2 cup roasted red peppers.
- ✓ 2 tablespoons tahini
- ✓ 2 cloves garlic, minced.
- ✓ 2 tablespoons lemon juice
- ✓ 2 tablespoons olive oil
- ✓ Salt and pepper to taste

Instructions:

1. Combine all ingredients in the slow cooker.
2. Cook on low for 2 hours.
3. Blend until smooth using a blender or immersion blender.

Nutritional Information (per serving):

Calories: 120, Protein: 5g, Carbs: 15g, Fat: 5g, Fiber: 4g.

Slow Cooker Buffalo Cauliflower Bites

Cooking Time: 2 hours

Serving: 4

Ingredients:

- ✓ 1 head cauliflower, cut into florets.
- ✓ 1/2 cup hot sauce
- ✓ 2 tablespoons low-fat butter or margarine
- ✓ 1 teaspoon garlic powder
- ✓ Salt and pepper to taste

Instructions:

1. Place cauliflower florets in the slow cooker.
2. In a bowl, mix hot sauce, butter, garlic powder, salt, and pepper.
3. Pour the mixture over the cauliflower.
4. Cook on low for 2 hours.

Nutritional Information (per serving):

Calories: 90, Protein: 3g, Carbs: 10g, Fat: 5g, Fiber: 3g.

Slow Cooker Caprese Skewers

Cooking Time: 1 hour

Serving: 8

Ingredients:

- ✓ 16 small fresh mozzarella balls
- ✓ 16 cherry tomatoes
- ✓ 16 fresh basil leaves
- ✓ 2 tablespoons balsamic glaze
- ✓ Salt and pepper to taste

Instructions:

1. Thread mozzarella balls, cherry tomatoes, and basil leaves onto skewers.
2. Place skewers in the slow cooker.
3. Drizzle with balsamic glaze, salt, and pepper.
4. Cook on low for 1 hour.

Nutritional Information (per serving):

Calories: 80, Protein: 4g, Carbs: 3g, Fat: 5g, Fiber: 1g.

Slow Cooker Spiced Nuts

Cooking Time: 2 hours

Serving: 10

Ingredients:

- ✓ 2 cups mixed nuts (almonds, pecans, walnuts)
- ✓ 1/4 cup maple syrup
- ✓ 1 teaspoon ground cinnamon
- ✓ 1/2 teaspoon ground nutmeg
- ✓ 1/2 teaspoon cayenne pepper
- ✓ Salt to taste

Instructions:

1. Place mixed nuts in the slow cooker.
2. In a bowl, mix maple syrup, cinnamon, nutmeg, cayenne pepper, and salt.
3. Pour the mixture over the nuts.
4. Cook on low for 2 hours, stirring occasionally.

Nutritional Information (per serving):

Calories: 170, Protein: 5g, Carbs: 11g, Fat: 12g, Fiber: 2g.

Slow Cooker Greek Yogurt and Cucumber Dip

Cooking Time: 2 hours

Serving: 6

Ingredients:

- ✓ 2 cups low-fat Greek yogurt
- ✓ 1 cucumber grated and drained.
- ✓ 2 cloves garlic, minced.
- ✓ 2 tablespoons fresh dill, chopped.
- ✓ Salt and pepper to taste

Instructions:

1. Combine Greek yogurt, grated cucumber, garlic, dill, salt, and pepper in the slow cooker.
2. Cook on low for 2 hours, stirring occasionally.

Nutritional Information (per serving):

Calories: 80, Protein: 7g, Carbs: 8g, Fat: 2g, Fiber: 1g.

Slow Cooker Stuffed Mushrooms

Cooking Time: 3 hours

Serving: 6

Ingredients:

- ✓ 18 large mushroom caps
- ✓ 1/2 cup breadcrumbs
- ✓ 1/4 cup grated Parmesan cheese
- ✓ 2 cloves garlic, minced.
- ✓ 2 tablespoons fresh parsley, chopped.
- ✓ Salt and pepper to taste

Instructions:

1. Remove stems from mushroom caps.
2. In a bowl, mix breadcrumbs, Parmesan, garlic, parsley, salt, and pepper.
3. Stuff mushroom caps with the breadcrumb mixture.
4. **Place in the slow cooker and cook on low for 3 hours.**

Nutritional Information (per serving):

Calories: 80, Protein: 4g, Carbs: 8g, Fat: 4g, Fiber: 1g.

Slow Cooker Fruit Compote

Cooking Time: 2 hours

Serving: 8

Ingredients:

- ✓ 4 cups mixed fruit (e.g., apples, pears, berries)
- ✓ 1/4 cup honey
- ✓ 1 teaspoon vanilla extract
- ✓ 1/2 teaspoon ground cinnamon

Instructions:

1. Combine mixed fruit, honey, vanilla extract, and ground cinnamon in the slow cooker.
2. Cook on low for 2 hours, stirring occasionally.

Nutritional Information (per serving):

Calories: 80, Protein: 1g, Carbs: 20g, Fat: 0g, Fiber: 3g.

Slow Cooker Roasted Garlic and White Bean Dip

Cooking Time: 2 hours

Serving: 8

Ingredients:

- ✓ 2 cans (15 oz each) white beans, drained and rinsed.
- ✓ 1 bulb roasted garlic.
- ✓ 2 tablespoons lemon juice
- ✓ 2 tablespoons olive oil
- ✓ 1/2 teaspoon smoked paprika.
- ✓ Salt and pepper to taste

Instructions:

1. Combine white beans, roasted garlic, lemon juice, olive oil, smoked paprika, salt, and pepper in the slow cooker.
2. Cook on low for 2 hours.
3. Blend until smooth using a blender or immersion blender.

Nutritional Information (per serving):

Calories: 110, Protein: 5g, Carbs: 18g, Fat: 2g, Fiber: 4g.

Chapter 7

Desserts and Treats

Slow Cooker Apple Cinnamon Oatmeal

Cooking Time: 2 hours

Serving: 4

Ingredients:

- ✓ 1 cup steel-cut oats
- ✓ 4 cups unsweetened apple juice
- ✓ 2 apples peeled and chopped.
- ✓ 1 teaspoon ground cinnamon
- ✓ 1/4 cup honey
- ✓ 1/4 cup chopped nuts (optional)

Instructions:

1. Combine oats, apple juice, apples, and cinnamon in the slow cooker.
2. Cook on low for 2 hours, stirring occasionally.
3. Drizzle with honey and sprinkle with nuts before serving.

Nutritional Information (per serving):

Calories: 300, Protein: 6g, Carbs: 65g, Fat: 5g, Fiber: 7g.

Slow Cooker Rice Pudding

Cooking Time: 2 hours

Serving: 6

Ingredients:

- ✓ 1 cup arborio rice
- ✓ 4 cups low-fat milk
- ✓ 1/2 cup sugar
- ✓ 1 teaspoon vanilla extract
- ✓ 1/2 teaspoon ground cinnamon
- ✓ 1/4 teaspoon ground nutmeg
- ✓ Raisins and chopped nuts for garnish (optional)

Instructions:

1. Combine rice, milk, sugar, vanilla, cinnamon, and nutmeg in the slow cooker.
2. Cook on low for 2 hours, stirring occasionally.
3. Garnish with raisins and chopped nuts if desired before serving.

Nutritional Information (per serving):

Calories: 250, Protein: 6g, Carbs: 50g, Fat: 2g, Fiber: 1g.

Slow Cooker Berry Cobbler

Cooking Time: 3 hours

Serving: 6

Ingredients:

- ✓ 3 cups mixed berries (strawberries, blueberries, raspberries)
- ✓ 1/2 cup sugar
- ✓ 1 cup all-purpose flour
- ✓ 1 teaspoon baking powder
- ✓ 1/2 cup low-fat milk
- ✓ 1/4 cup low-fat butter or margarine

Instructions:

1. In a bowl, mix mixed berries and sugar, then transfer to the slow cooker.
2. In another bowl, combine flour, baking powder, milk, and melted butter.
3. Pour the batter over the berries in the slow cooker.
4. Cook on low for 3 hours.

Nutritional Information (per serving):

Calories: 250, Protein: 3g, Carbs: 50g, Fat: 3g, Fiber: 4g.

Slow Cooker Banana Bread

Cooking Time: 2 hours

Serving: 8

Ingredients:

- ✓ 3 ripe bananas, mashed.
- ✓ 1/2 cup sugar
- ✓ 1/4 cup low-fat butter or margarine
- ✓ 1 teaspoon vanilla extract
- ✓ 2 cups all-purpose flour
- ✓ 1 teaspoon baking powder
- ✓ 1/2 teaspoon baking soda

Instructions:

1. In a bowl, mix mashed bananas, sugar, melted butter, and vanilla extract.
2. Stir in flour, baking powder, and baking soda.
3. Transfer the mixture to the slow cooker.
4. Cook on low for 2 hours.

Nutritional Information (per serving):

Calories: 270, Protein: 3g, Carbs: 55g, Fat: 5g, Fiber: 2g.

Slow Cooker Chocolate Pudding Cake

Cooking Time: 2 hours

Serving: 6

Ingredients:

- ✓ 1 cup all-purpose flour
- ✓ 3/4 cup sugar
- ✓ 2 tablespoons unsweetened cocoa powder
- ✓ 2 teaspoons baking powder
- ✓ 1/4 teaspoon salt
- ✓ 1/2 cup low-fat milk
- ✓ 2 tablespoons cocoa powder (for the topping)
- ✓ 1 cup hot water

Instructions:

1. In a bowl, combine flour, 1/2 cup sugar, 2 tablespoons cocoa powder, baking powder, and salt.
2. Stir in milk and mix until smooth. Pour the mixture into the slow cooker.
3. In a separate bowl, mix 1/4 cup sugar and 2 tablespoons cocoa powder. Sprinkle this mixture over the batter.
4. Pour hot water over the top. Do not stir.
5. Cook on low for 2 hours.

Nutritional Information (per serving):

Calories: 260, Protein: 4g, Carbs: 60g, Fat: 2g, Fiber: 3g.

Slow Cooker Poached Pears

Cooking Time: 2 hours

Serving: 4

Ingredients:

- ✓ 4 ripe pears peeled and cored.
- ✓ 2 cups unsweetened apple juice
- ✓ 1/2 cup sugar
- ✓ 1 cinnamon stick
- ✓ 1 teaspoon vanilla extract

Instructions:

1. Place pears in the slow cooker.
2. In a bowl, mix apple juice, sugar, cinnamon stick, and vanilla extract. Pour over the pears.
3. Cook on low for 2 hours.

Nutritional Information (per serving):

Calories: 200, Protein: 1g, Carbs: 50g, Fat: 0g, Fiber: 6g.

Slow Cooker Peach Crisp

Cooking Time: 3 hours

Serving: 6

Ingredients:

- ✓ 4 cups sliced peaches (fresh or frozen)
- ✓ 1/2 cup sugar
- ✓ 1/2 cup oats
- ✓ 1/4 cup all-purpose flour
- ✓ 1/4 cup low-fat butter or margarine
- ✓ 1/2 teaspoon ground cinnamon

Instructions:

1. Place sliced peaches in the slow cooker.
2. In a bowl, combine sugar, oats, flour, melted butter, and cinnamon. Sprinkle over the peaches.
3. Cook on low for 3 hours.

Nutritional Information (per serving):

Calories: 250, Protein: 2g, Carbs: 50g, Fat: 6g, Fiber: 3g.

Slow Cooker Lemon Berry Cheesecake

Cooking Time: 2 hours

Serving: 8

Ingredients:

- ✓ 1 cup graham cracker crumbs
- ✓ 2 tablespoons low-fat butter or margarine
- ✓ 8 oz low-fat cream cheese
- ✓ 1/2 cup sugar
- ✓ 2 eggs
- ✓ 1/2 cup low-fat Greek yogurt
- ✓ Zest and juice of 1 lemon
- ✓ 1 cup mixed berries (strawberries, blueberries, raspberries)

Instructions:

1. In a bowl, combine graham cracker crumbs and melted butter. Press into the bottom of the slow cooker.
2. In another bowl, beat cream cheese, sugar, eggs, Greek yogurt, lemon zest, and lemon juice until smooth.
3. Pour the cream cheese mixture over the crust.
4. Cook on low for 2 hours.
5. Top with mixed berries before serving.

Nutritional Information (per serving):

Calories: 220, Protein: 7g, Carbs: 28g, Fat: 8g, Fiber: 2g.

Slow Cooker Chocolate Fondue

Cooking Time: 1 hour

Serving: 6

Ingredients:

- ✓ 1 cup semi-sweet chocolate chips
- ✓ 1/2 cup low-fat milk
- ✓ 1 teaspoon vanilla extract
- ✓ Assorted dippers (strawberries, banana slices, marshmallows, pretzels)

Instructions:

1. In the slow cooker, combine chocolate chips, milk, and vanilla extract.
2. Cook on low for 1 hour, stirring occasionally.
3. Serve with assorted dippers for fondue.

Nutritional Information (per serving):

Calories: 200, Protein: 2g, Carbs: 30g, Fat: 8g, Fiber: 3g.

Slow Cooker Pumpkin Pie Pudding

Cooking Time: 2 hours

Serving: 6

Ingredients:

- ✓ 1 can (15 oz) pumpkin puree
- ✓ 1/2 cup sugar
- ✓ 1/2 cup low-fat milk
- ✓ 2 eggs
- ✓ 1 teaspoon vanilla extract
- ✓ 1/2 teaspoon ground cinnamon
- ✓ 1/4 teaspoon ground nutmeg
- ✓ 1/4 teaspoon ground ginger
- ✓ Whipped cream for garnish (optional)

Instructions:

1. In a bowl, whisk together pumpkin puree, sugar, milk, eggs, vanilla extract, and spices.
2. Pour the mixture into the slow cooker.
3. Cook on low for 2 hours.
4. Serve warm, garnished with whipped cream if desired.

Nutritional Information (per serving):

Calories: 180, Protein: 5g, Carbs: 30g, Fat: 5g, Fiber: 3g.

Chapter 8

Beverages and Smoothies

Slow Cooker Spiced Apple Cider

Cooking Time: 4 hours

Serving: 8

Ingredients:

- ✓ 8 cups unsweetened apple cider
- ✓ 4 cinnamon sticks
- ✓ 6 whole cloves
- ✓ 1 orange, sliced.
- ✓ 1/4 cup honey (optional)

Instructions:

1. Combine apple cider, cinnamon sticks, cloves, and orange slices in the slow cooker.
2. Cook on low for 4 hours.
3. Add honey if desired and stir before serving.

Nutritional Information (per serving):

Calories: 120, Carbs: 30g, Fat: 0g.

Slow Cooker Hot Chocolate

Cooking Time: 2 hours

Serving: 6

Ingredients:

- ✓ 6 cups low-fat milk
- ✓ 1 cup semi-sweet chocolate chips
- ✓ 1/4 cup unsweetened cocoa powder
- ✓ 1/4 cup sugar
- ✓ 1 teaspoon vanilla extract
- ✓ Pinch of salt

Instructions:

1. In the slow cooker, combine milk, chocolate chips, cocoa powder, sugar, vanilla, and salt.
2. Cook on low for 2 hours, stirring occasionally.
3. Serve hot.

Nutritional Information (per serving):

Calories: 220, Protein: 7g, Carbs: 33g, Fat: 8g, Fiber: 3g.

Slow Cooker Ginger Turmeric Tea

Cooking Time: 2 hours

Serving: 4

Ingredients:

- ✓ 4 cups water
- ✓ 1-inch piece of fresh ginger, sliced
- ✓ 1-inch piece of fresh turmeric, sliced (or 1 teaspoon ground turmeric)
- ✓ 1 lemon, sliced.
- ✓ Honey to taste

Instructions:

1. In the slow cooker, combine water, ginger, turmeric, and lemon slices.
2. Cook on low for 2 hours.
3. Add honey to taste and serve warm.

Nutritional Information (per serving):

Calories: 5, Carbs: 1g, Fat: 0g.

Slow Cooker Green Tea with Mint and Honey

Cooking Time: 1 hour

Serving: 4

Ingredients:

- ✓ 4 cups water
- ✓ 4 green tea bags
- ✓ 1/4 cup fresh mint leaves
- ✓ Honey to taste

Instructions:

1. In the slow cooker, combine water, green tea bags, and mint leaves.
2. Cook on low for 1 hour.
3. Add honey to taste and serve hot or over ice.

Nutritional Information (per serving):

Calories: 0, Carbs: 0g, Fat: 0g.

Slow Cooker Mango Lassi

Cooking Time: 2 hours

Serving: 4

Ingredients:

- ✓ 2 cups low-fat yogurt
- ✓ 2 cups ripe mango chunks (fresh or frozen)
- ✓ 1/4 cup sugar (adjust to taste)
- ✓ 1/2 teaspoon ground cardamom
- ✓ Ice cubes (optional)

Instructions:

1. Blend the yogurt, mango chunks, sugar, and cardamom until smooth.
2. Pour the mixture into the slow cooker.
3. Cook on low for 2 hours.
4. Serve chilled with ice cubes if desired.

Nutritional Information (per serving):

Calories: 180, Protein: 5g, Carbs: 40g, Fat: 1g.

Slow Cooker Beet and Berry Smoothie

Cooking Time: 1 hour

Serving: 4

Ingredients:

- ✓ 2 medium beets peeled and chopped.
- ✓ 2 cups mixed berries (strawberries, blueberries, raspberries)
- ✓ 1 cup low-fat yogurt
- ✓ 1 tablespoon honey
- ✓ 1 cup water

Instructions:

1. Combine beets, mixed berries, yogurt, honey, and water in the slow cooker.
2. Cook on low for 1 hour.
3. Blend until smooth and serve.

Nutritional Information (per serving):

Calories: 120, Protein: 4g, Carbs: 25g, Fat: 1g, Fiber: 5g.

Slow Cooker Cranberry Orange Punch

Cooking Time: 2 hours

Serving: 8

Ingredients:

- ✓ 4 cups unsweetened cranberry juice
- ✓ 2 cups orange juice
- ✓ 1 cup pineapple juice
- ✓ 1/4 cup honey
- ✓ 1 orange, sliced.
- ✓ 1 lemon, sliced.

Instructions:

1. Combine cranberry juice, orange juice, pineapple juice, honey, orange slices, and lemon slices in the slow cooker.
2. Cook on low for 2 hours.
3. Serve warm or chilled.

Nutritional Information (per serving):

Calories: 90, Carbs: 24g, Fat: 0g.

Slow Cooker Strawberry Kiwi Smoothie

Cooking Time: 1 hour

Serving: 4

Ingredients:

- ✓ 2 cups strawberries (fresh or frozen)
- ✓ 2 kiwis peeled and sliced.
- ✓ 2 cups low-fat yogurt
- ✓ 2 tablespoons honey
- ✓ 1 cup water

Instructions:

1. Combine strawberries, kiwis, yogurt, honey, and water in the slow cooker.
2. Cook on low for 1 hour.
3. Blend until smooth and serve.

Nutritional Information (per serving):

Calories: 160, Protein: 5g, Carbs: 35g, Fat: 1g, Fiber: 4g.

Slow Cooker Iced Chai Tea Latte

Cooking Time: 2 hours

Serving: 4

Ingredients:

- ✓ 4 cups water
- ✓ 4 chai tea bags
- ✓ 1 cup low-fat milk
- ✓ 2 tablespoons honey
- ✓ Ice cubes

Instructions:

1. In the slow cooker, combine water and chai tea bags.
2. Cook on low for 2 hours.
3. Remove tea bags and stir in milk and honey.
4. Serve over ice.

Nutritional Information (per serving):

Calories: 60, Protein: 2g, Carbs: 12g, Fat: 1g.

Slow Cooker Pineapple Coconut Smoothie

Cooking Time: 1 hour

Serving: 4

Ingredients:

- ✓ 2 cups pineapple chunks
- ✓ 1 cup coconut milk
- ✓ 1 cup low-fat yogurt
- ✓ 2 tablespoons honey
- ✓ 1 cup ice cubes

Instructions:

1. Combine pineapple chunks, coconut milk, yogurt, honey, and ice cubes in the slow cooker.
2. Cook on low for 1 hour.
3. Blend until smooth and serve.

Nutritional Information (per serving):

Calories: 180, Protein: 3g, Carbs: 25g, Fat: 8g, Fiber: 2g.

Chapter 9

28-Day Meal Plan

Day	Breakfast	Lunch	Dinner	Snacks	Beverages
Day 1	Slow Cooker Oatmeal	Slow Cooker Hearty Vegetable Soup	Slow Cooker Lemon Herb Chicken	Mixed Nuts	Slow Cooker Spiced Apple Cider
Day 2	Slow Cooker Greek Yogurt and Cucumber Dip	Slow Cooker Wild Rice and Mushroom Pilaf	Slow Cooker Sweet Potato and Lentil Curry	Baby Carrots with Hummus	Slow Cooker Chocolate Fondue
Day 3	Slow Cooker Salsa Verde Chicken Wings	Slow Cooker Quinoa and Black Bean Salad	Slow Cooker Nutrient-Rich Beef Stew	Slow Cooker Berry Cobbler	Slow Cooker Mango Lassi
Day 4	Slow Cooker Roasted Red	Slow Cooker Caprese Skewers	Slow Cooker Balsamic Glazed Chicken	Slow Cooker Spiced Nuts	Slow Cooker Ginger Turmeric Tea

	Pepper Hummus				
Day 5	Slow Cooker Roasted Garlic and White Bean Dip	Slow Cooker Fruit Compote	Slow Cooker Mediterranean Chicken Thighs	Mixed Berries	Slow Cooker Hot Chocolate
Day 6	Slow Cooker Spinach and Artichoke Dip	Slow Cooker Stuffed Mushrooms	Slow Cooker Turkey and Vegetable Soup	Mixed Nuts	Slow Cooker Cranberry Orange Punch
Day 7	Slow Cooker Wild Rice and Mushroom Pilaf	Slow Cooker Greek Yogurt and Cucumber Dip	Slow Cooker Roasted Vegetable Ratatouille	Baby Carrots with Hummus	Slow Cooker Green Tea with Mint and Honey
Day 8	Slow Cooker Banana Bread	Slow Cooker Quinoa and Black Bean Salad	Slow Cooker Lemon Herb Chicken	Slow Cooker Roasted Red Pepper Hummus	Slow Cooker Strawberry Kiwi Smoothie

Day 9	Slow Cooker Roasted Red Pepper Hummus	Slow Cooker Salsa Verde Chicken Wings	Slow Cooker Sweet Potato and Lentil Curry	Mixed Berries	Slow Cooker Spiced Apple Cider
Day 10	Slow Cooker Caprese Skewers	Slow Cooker Caprese Skewers	Slow Cooker Balsamic Glazed Chicken	Mixed Nuts	Slow Cooker Iced Chai Tea Latte
Day 11	Slow Cooker Salsa Verde Chicken Wings	Slow Cooker Nutrient-Rich Beef Stew	Slow Cooker Mediterranean Chicken Thighs	Baby Carrots with Hummus	Slow Cooker Chocolate Fondue
Day 12	Slow Cooker Greek Yogurt and Cucumber Dip	Slow Cooker Wild Rice and Mushroom Pilaf	Slow Cooker Roasted Vegetable Ratatouille	Slow Cooker Berry Cobbler	Slow Cooker Pineapple Coconut Smoothie
Day 13	Slow Cooker Banana Bread	Slow Cooker Quinoa and Black Bean Salad	Slow Cooker Lemon Herb Chicken	Mixed Berries	Slow Cooker Hot Chocolate

Day 14	Slow Cooker Roasted Garlic and White Bean Dip	Slow Cooker Fruit Compote	Slow Cooker Sweet Potato and Lentil Curry	Mixed Nuts	Slow Cooker Ginger Turmeric Tea
Day 15	Slow Cooker Spinach and Artichoke Dip	Slow Cooker Stuffed Mushrooms	Slow Cooker Balsamic Glazed Chicken	Baby Carrots with Hummus	Slow Cooker Mango Lassi
Day 16	Slow Cooker Wild Rice and Mushroom Pilaf	Slow Cooker Caprese Skewers	Slow Cooker Mediterranean Chicken Thighs	Mixed Berries	Slow Cooker Cranberry Orange Punch
Day 17	Slow Cooker Salsa Verde Chicken Wings	Slow Cooker Greek Yogurt and Cucumber Dip	Slow Cooker Roasted Vegetable Ratatouille	Mixed Nuts	Slow Cooker Green Tea with Mint and Honey
Day 18	Slow Cooker Roasted	Slow Cooker	Slow Cooker Lemon Herb Chicken	Slow Cooker Roasted	Slow Cooker Strawberry

				Red Pepper Hummus	Banana Bread		Red Pepper Hummus	Kiwi Smoothie
Day 19	Slow Cooker Caprese Skewers	Slow Cooker Quinoa and Black Bean Salad	Slow Cooker Sweet Potato and Lentil Curry	Baby Carrots with Hummus	Slow Cooker Spiced Apple Cider
Day 20	Slow Cooker Salsa Verde Chicken Wings	Slow Cooker Nutrient-Rich Beef Stew	Slow Cooker Balsamic Glazed Chicken	Mixed Berries	Slow Cooker Chocolate Fondue
Day 21	Slow Cooker Greek Yogurt and Cucumber Dip	Slow Cooker Wild Rice and Mushroom Pilaf	Slow Cooker Mediterranean Chicken Thighs	Mixed Nuts	Slow Cooker Hot Chocolate
Day 22	Slow Cooker Roasted Garlic and White Bean Dip	Slow Cooker Fruit Compote	Slow Cooker Roasted Vegetable Ratatouille	Mixed Berries	Slow Cooker Ginger Turmeric Tea

Day 23	Slow Cooker Spinach and Artichoke Dip	Slow Cooker Stuffed Mushrooms	Slow Cooker Lemon Herb Chicken	Baby Carrots with Hummus	Slow Cooker Mango Lassi
Day 24	Slow Cooker Wild Rice and Mushroom Pilaf	Slow Cooker Caprese Skewers	Slow Cooker Sweet Potato and Lentil Curry	Mixed Nuts	Slow Cooker Iced Chai Tea Latte
Day 25	Slow Cooker Banana Bread	Slow Cooker Quinoa and Black Bean Salad	Slow Cooker Mediterranean Chicken Thighs	Baby Carrots with Hummus	Slow Cooker Spiced Apple Cider
Day 26	Slow Cooker Roasted Red Pepper Hummus	Slow Cooker Caprese Skewers	Slow Cooker Balsamic Glazed Chicken	Mixed Berries	Slow Cooker Strawberry Kiwi Smoothie
Day 27	Slow Cooker Salsa Verde	Slow Cooker Nutrient-	Slow Cooker Roasted Vegetable Ratatouille	Mixed Nuts	Slow Cooker Cranberry

	Chicken Wings	Rich Beef Stew			Orange Punch
Day 28	Slow Cooker Greek Yogurt and Cucumber Dip	Slow Cooker Fruit Compote	Slow Cooker Lemon Herb Chicken	Slow Cooker Berry Cobbler	Slow Cooker Pineapple Coconut Smoothie

CONCLUSION

In closing, our journey of healing and hope has been a testament to the extraordinary power of food, love, and resilience. The slow cooker cirrhosis diet cookbook that we have crafted together is not just a collection of recipes; it is a lifeline, a bridge from despair to optimism, and a symbol of the unwavering strength that resides within us all.

Through the trials and tribulations of cirrhosis, we discovered that food can be more than sustenance; it can be a source of comfort, pleasure, and even transformation. The slow cooker became our ally, gently coaxing out the flavors of fresh ingredients and weaving them into dishes that could inspire anyone to embark on a journey of healing.

This cookbook is our gift to you, a beacon of light in the sometimes dark and uncertain world of liver disease. Whether you're a patient bravely battling cirrhosis, a dedicated caregiver, or a concerned friend, we invite you to embrace these recipes and make them a part of your life. Let the tantalizing aromas and delectable flavors nourish your body and spirit, just as they did for us.

As we stand at the threshold of a new chapter in your life, remember that you are not alone. We have walked this path, faced the challenges, and celebrated the victories together. The slow cooker cirrhosis diet cookbook is a testament to the power of community, support, and the resilience of the human spirit.

Our hope is that this book becomes a source of inspiration, a source of comfort, and a source of determination for all those who are confronted by cirrhosis or any health challenge. May it remind you that even in the most trying times, there is always a glimmer of hope, a moment of joy, and a reason to keep moving forward.

We are living proof that with the right nourishment, the right mindset, and the right support, miracles can happen. Just as Emily's health improved and her spirit rekindled, so too can your journey take a turn for the better. The recipes within these pages are more than just ingredients and instructions; they are a promise of better days to come, of renewed vitality, and of the possibility of a brighter tomorrow.

So, with that, we bid you farewell on this chapter of our journey. Thank you for sharing in our story, and we hope that you find comfort, healing, and hope within these pages. May you embark on your own journey of transformation, just as we did, and may these recipes be the guiding stars on your path to wellness.

Remember, you are not alone, and there is always a glimmer of hope, even in the darkest of times. Embrace the power of food, love, and resilience, and let it carry you toward a healthier, happier future. You have the strength within you, and these recipes are here to light your way.

With heartfelt gratitude and warmest wishes for your journey ahead.

MEAL PLANNER JOURNAL

CIRRHOSIS MEAL JOURNAL PLANNER

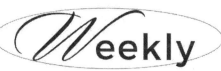

WEEK _____   MONTH _____

MONDAY
BREAKFAST
LUNCH
SNACK
DINNER

TUESDAY
BREAKFAST
LUNCH
SNACK
DINNER

WEDNESDAY
BREAKFAST
LUNCH
SNACK
DINNER

THURSDAY
BREAKFAST
LUNCH
SNACK
DINNER

FRIDAY
BREAKFAST
LUNCH
SNACK
DINNER

SATURDAY
BREAKFAST
LUNCH
SNACK
DINNER

SUNDAY
BREAKFAST
LUNCH
SNACK
DINNER

SHOPPING LIST
- ○ _____
- ○ _____
- ○ _____
- ○ _____
- ○ _____
- ○ _____
- ○ _____

NOTE

CIRRHOSIS MEAL JOURNAL PLANNER

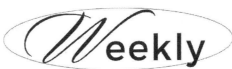

WEEK _____   MONTH _____

MONDAY
BREAKFAST
LUNCH
SNACK
DINNER

TUESDAY
BREAKFAST
LUNCH
SNACK
DINNER

WEDNESDAY
BREAKFAST
LUNCH
SNACK
DINNER

THURSDAY
BREAKFAST
LUNCH
SNACK
DINNER

FRIDAY
BREAKFAST
LUNCH
SNACK
DINNER

SATURDAY
BREAKFAST
LUNCH
SNACK
DINNER

SUNDAY
BREAKFAST
LUNCH
SNACK
DINNER

SHOPPING LIST
- ○ _____
- ○ _____
- ○ _____
- ○ _____
- ○ _____
- ○ _____
- ○ _____

NOTE

CIRRHOSIS MEAL JOURNAL PLANNER

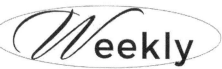

WEEK _____   MONTH _____

MONDAY
BREAKFAST
LUNCH
SNACK
DINNER

TUESDAY
BREAKFAST
LUNCH
SNACK
DINNER

WEDNESDAY
BREAKFAST
LUNCH
SNACK
DINNER

THURSDAY
BREAKFAST
LUNCH
SNACK
DINNER

FRIDAY
BREAKFAST
LUNCH
SNACK
DINNER

SATURDAY
BREAKFAST
LUNCH
SNACK
DINNER

SUNDAY
BREAKFAST
LUNCH
SNACK
DINNER

SHOPPING LIST
- _____
- _____
- _____
- _____
- _____
- _____
- _____

NOTE

CIRRHOSIS MEAL JOURNAL PLANNER

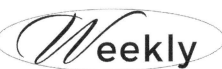

WEEK _____   MONTH _____

MONDAY
BREAKFAST
LUNCH
SNACK
DINNER

TUESDAY
BREAKFAST
LUNCH
SNACK
DINNER

WEDNESDAY
BREAKFAST
LUNCH
SNACK
DINNER

THURSDAY
BREAKFAST
LUNCH
SNACK
DINNER

FRIDAY
BREAKFAST
LUNCH
SNACK
DINNER

SATURDAY
BREAKFAST
LUNCH
SNACK
DINNER

SUNDAY
BREAKFAST
LUNCH
SNACK
DINNER

SHOPPING LIST
- ○ _____
- ○ _____
- ○ _____
- ○ _____
- ○ _____
- ○ _____
- ○ _____

NOTE

CIRRHOSIS MEAL JOURNAL PLANNER

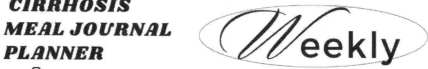

WEEK _____   MONTH _____

MONDAY
BREAKFAST
LUNCH
SNACK
DINNER

TUESDAY
BREAKFAST
LUNCH
SNACK
DINNER

WEDNESDAY
BREAKFAST
LUNCH
SNACK
DINNER

THURSDAY
BREAKFAST
LUNCH
SNACK
DINNER

FRIDAY
BREAKFAST
LUNCH
SNACK
DINNER

SATURDAY
BREAKFAST
LUNCH
SNACK
DINNER

SUNDAY
BREAKFAST
LUNCH
SNACK
DINNER

SHOPPING LIST
○ _____
○ _____
○ _____
○ _____
○ _____
○ _____
○ _____

NOTE

CIRRHOSIS MEAL JOURNAL PLANNER

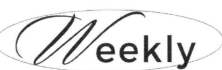

WEEK _____   MONTH _____

MONDAY
BREAKFAST
LUNCH
SNACK
DINNER

TUESDAY
BREAKFAST
LUNCH
SNACK
DINNER

WEDNESDAY
BREAKFAST
LUNCH
SNACK
DINNER

THURSDAY
BREAKFAST
LUNCH
SNACK
DINNER

FRIDAY
BREAKFAST
LUNCH
SNACK
DINNER

SATURDAY
BREAKFAST
LUNCH
SNACK
DINNER

SUNDAY
BREAKFAST
LUNCH
SNACK
DINNER

SHOPPING LIST
- ○ _____
- ○ _____
- ○ _____
- ○ _____
- ○ _____
- ○ _____
- ○ _____

NOTE

CIRRHOSIS MEAL JOURNAL PLANNER

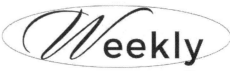

WEEK _____   MONTH _____

MONDAY
BREAKFAST
LUNCH
SNACK
DINNER

TUESDAY
BREAKFAST
LUNCH
SNACK
DINNER

WEDNESDAY
BREAKFAST
LUNCH
SNACK
DINNER

THURSDAY
BREAKFAST
LUNCH
SNACK
DINNER

FRIDAY
BREAKFAST
LUNCH
SNACK
DINNER

SATURDAY
BREAKFAST
LUNCH
SNACK
DINNER

SUNDAY
BREAKFAST
LUNCH
SNACK
DINNER

SHOPPING LIST
○ _____
○ _____
○ _____
○ _____
○ _____
○ _____
○ _____

NOTE

CIRRHOSIS MEAL JOURNAL PLANNER

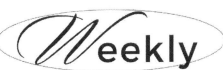

WEEK _____   MONTH _____

MONDAY
BREAKFAST
LUNCH
SNACK
DINNER

TUESDAY
BREAKFAST
LUNCH
SNACK
DINNER

WEDNESDAY
BREAKFAST
LUNCH
SNACK
DINNER

THURSDAY
BREAKFAST
LUNCH
SNACK
DINNER

FRIDAY
BREAKFAST
LUNCH
SNACK
DINNER

SATURDAY
BREAKFAST
LUNCH
SNACK
DINNER

SUNDAY
BREAKFAST
LUNCH
SNACK
DINNER

SHOPPING LIST
- _____
- _____
- _____
- _____
- _____
- _____
- _____

NOTE

CIRRHOSIS MEAL JOURNAL PLANNER

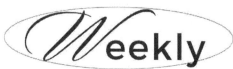

WEEK _____

MONTH _____

MONDAY
BREAKFAST
LUNCH
SNACK
DINNER

TUESDAY
BREAKFAST
LUNCH
SNACK
DINNER

WEDNESDAY
BREAKFAST
LUNCH
SNACK
DINNER

THURSDAY
BREAKFAST
LUNCH
SNACK
DINNER

FRIDAY
BREAKFAST
LUNCH
SNACK
DINNER

SATURDAY
BREAKFAST
LUNCH
SNACK
DINNER

SUNDAY
BREAKFAST
LUNCH
SNACK
DINNER

SHOPPING LIST
- ○ _____
- ○ _____
- ○ _____
- ○ _____
- ○ _____
- ○ _____
- ○ _____

NOTE

CIRRHOSIS MEAL JOURNAL PLANNER

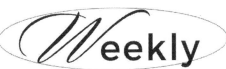

WEEK _____ MONTH ....

MONDAY
BREAKFAST
LUNCH
SNACK
DINNER

TUESDAY
BREAKFAST
LUNCH
SNACK
DINNER

WEDNESDAY
BREAKFAST
LUNCH
SNACK
DINNER

THURSDAY
BREAKFAST
LUNCH
SNACK
DINNER

FRIDAY
BREAKFAST
LUNCH
SNACK
DINNER

SATURDAY
BREAKFAST
LUNCH
SNACK
DINNER

SUNDAY
BREAKFAST
LUNCH
SNACK
DINNER

SHOPPING LIST
- ○ _____
- ○ _____
- ○ _____
- ○ _____
- ○ _____
- ○ _____
- ○ _____

NOTE

CIRRHOSIS MEAL JOURNAL PLANNER

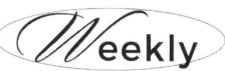

WEEK _____   MONTH _____

MONDAY
BREAKFAST
LUNCH
SNACK
DINNER

TUESDAY
BREAKFAST
LUNCH
SNACK
DINNER

WEDNESDAY
BREAKFAST
LUNCH
SNACK
DINNER

THURSDAY
BREAKFAST
LUNCH
SNACK
DINNER

FRIDAY
BREAKFAST
LUNCH
SNACK
DINNER

SATURDAY
BREAKFAST
LUNCH
SNACK
DINNER

SUNDAY
BREAKFAST
LUNCH
SNACK
DINNER

SHOPPING LIST
- ○ _____
- ○ _____
- ○ _____
- ○ _____
- ○ _____
- ○ _____
- ○ _____

NOTE

CIRRHOSIS MEAL JOURNAL PLANNER

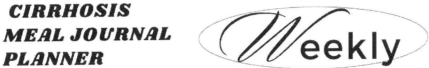

WEEK _____   **MONTH** _____

MONDAY

BREAKFAST

LUNCH

SNACK

DINNER

TUESDAY

BREAKFAST

LUNCH

SNACK

DINNER

WEDNESDAY

BREAKFAST

LUNCH

SNACK

DINNER

THURSDAY

BREAKFAST

LUNCH

SNACK

DINNER

FRIDAY

BREAKFAST

LUNCH

SNACK

DINNER

SATURDAY

BREAKFAST

LUNCH

SNACK

DINNER

SUNDAY

BREAKFAST

LUNCH

SNACK

DINNER

SHOPPING LIST

- ○ _____
- ○ _____
- ○ _____
- ○ _____
- ○ _____
- ○ _____
- ○ _____

NOTE

Made in United States
Orlando, FL
04 October 2024

52313554R00059